# "The Fast Feed and Repeat: Your Ultimate Guide to Delay and Avoid Denied Fasting Intermittently - Includes a Thirty-Day Fast Start."

By

Ella F. Miller

# Disclaimer

# Table of Content

# About The Author

Ella F. Miller is a dedicated supporter of holistic health and well-being. With considerable education and a belief in balance, she brings a wealth of skills to "The Fast Feed and Repeat".

Ella F. Miller has effectively assisted clients on their weight loss journeys, emphasizing self-awareness and self-compassion.

Her language is empathetic and transparent, making it easier to understand complicated health conditions. She's committed to giving a transforming approach to holistic health, enabling individuals to live happier, healthier lives.

Ella F. Miller continues to support conscious life and natural weight loss, urging individuals to appreciate life fully.

# Introduction

Welcome to "The Fast Feed and Repeat: Your Ultimate Guide to Delay and Avoid Denied Fasting Intermittently" - Include a Thirty-Day Fast Start." In this comprehensive guide, we embark on a transformative journey through the realms of intermittent fasting, exploring not only the art of delaying and avoiding denial but also the profound impact it can have on your health and well-being. Over the following pages, we'll dig into the nuances of intermittent fasting, comprehending its superiority over typical diets for weight loss, unraveling the health advantages that reach well beyond basic calorie reduction, and revealing the secrets underlying the 'Clean Fast.'

Our thirty-day Fast Start program is a guided entry into the world of intermittent fasting, fitting varied personality types and assuring a painless transition. From igniting your fast-burning superpower to understanding the scientifically-backed logic behind each tip, this book empowers you with the information to develop your unique intermittent fasting arsenal. Whether you're a newbie ready to begin your fasting adventure or a seasoned practitioner seeking refinement, "Fast. Feed, and Repeat" is your compass to sustainable fasting and lasting health. Let the journey begin.

**Unraveling the Superiority of Intermittent Fasting:**

**The Timing Paradigm:**

Intermittent fasting contradicts the common notion that lowering calories is the single path to weight reduction. By stressing the timing of meals, it taps into the body's inherent cycles, capitalizing on times of fasting to create a state of fat-burning. This tutorial elucidates how this subtle approach makes it unique from standard dieting strategies.

**The 'Clean Fast' Unveiled:**

At the center of intermittent fasting lies the notion of the 'Clean Fast.' It's not simply refraining from eating; it's a purposeful practice that maximizes the fasting state. Beyond the sheer avoidance of calorie intake, the 'Clean Fast' entails avoiding clear liquids and tastes. This section methodically explains the characteristics of a 'Clean Fast' and analyzes its vital role in unlocking the full potential of intermittent fasting.

**Navigating the Thirty-Day Fast Start:**

**Personalized Initiatives:**

Embarking on a thirty-day adventure, the Fast Start program is more than a set strategy; it's a tailored entry into the realm of intermittent fasting. Recognizing that people have various personalities and interests, this curriculum gives flexibility. From igniting the body's fat-burning capacity to progressively introducing different intermittent fasting patterns, it provides a smooth and personalized transition.

**Scientific Insight:**

This guide isn't simply a series of instructions; it's a window into the scientific logic behind each piece of advice. Readers get insight into the various mechanics that make intermittent fasting not simply a weight reduction method but a comprehensive approach to health. It looks into the physiological reactions, describing how fasting changes insulin levels, combats inflammation, and perhaps adds to lifespan.

**Beyond weight loss:**

**Extensive Health Benefits:**

While dropping pounds is a remarkable accomplishment, intermittent fasting's advantages extend well beyond weight reduction. It becomes a great ally in decreasing insulin levels, avoiding type 2 diabetes, and managing chronic inflammation. Supported by scientific research, this section explains how fasting may lead to a longer, healthier life by encouraging cellular processes like autophagy.

**Varied Fasting Styles Explored:**

Recognizing the variety of interests, this book exposes readers to numerous intermittent fasting strategies. From the commonly used 16:8 technique to the more rigorous OMAD approach, it permits people to pick a style that corresponds with their lifestyle. By giving alternatives and insights, it converts intermittent fasting into a sustainable and adaptive practice.

**Nourishing the Body for Lasting Health:**

**Synergy with Healthy Eating:**

Intermittent fasting is not a single treatment; it harmonizes with a balanced diet. This approach stresses the symbiotic link between fasting and replenishing the body with good meals. It investigates how fasting may transform your relationship with food, directing you towards healthier choices and restoring a natural balance to hunger signals.

**The Journey Unfolds:**

With "Fast, Feed, and Repeat" the journey into intermittent fasting becomes more than a lifestyle change; it's an educated experience. The book doesn't promise fast remedies but gives a thorough manual for change. Fast, feed, reaffirm—as the pages unfold, readers are prepared not just with practical tactics but with a deep grasp of the delicate dance between meal timing and enduring health.

# Chapter 1

# Fasting Unveiled: The Power of Meal Timing

## Introduction

The introductory chapter of "Fast, Feed, and Repeat" serves as a portal into the complicated realm of intermittent fasting by shining light on the transforming dynamics hidden in the scheduling of meals. This chapter is not only an introduction but also an investigation of how the strategic orchestration of eating windows may have a tremendous impact on weight control, general health, and the subtleties of metabolic processes.

**The Essence of Intermittent Fasting:**

Intermittent fasting stands as a deviation from standard weight control practices. This section navigates through the essence of intermittent fasting, demonstrating how it surpasses the typical emphasis on calorie intake. Emphasizing when one eats food, rather than just what or how much, leads readers to a paradigm shift in their view of dietary habits.

**Unraveling the Timing Paradigm:**

Delving further, this part unravels the core concepts of the timing paradigm within intermittent fasting. It explicates the complicated dance between mealtime and the body's internal systems. By investigating how various periods of eating and fasting affect insulin sensitivity, metabolic rate, and fat-burning mechanisms, readers get a comprehensive grasp of the physiological implications of strategic timing.

**The 'Clean Fast' Concept:**

Integral to the practice of intermittent fasting, the 'Clean Fast' notion takes center stage in this chapter. Moving beyond the sheer act of refraining from meals, it involves strategic tactics to keep the body in a fasting state optimally. This section painstakingly outlines what constitutes a 'Clean Fast,' incorporating not just food limits but also concerns for liquids and tastes that could disrupt the delicate balance of fasting.

**Scientific Basis of Meal Timing:**

This chapter further enhances the conversation by diving into the scientific basis of the focus on meal time. Readers go on a trip inside the complicated biochemistry of the body, gaining insights into how certain timing techniques impact hormone balance. Particularly, the research on insulin and ghrelin dynamics gives a scientific underpinning to the practical implementation of intermittent fasting.

**Cultural and Historical Perspectives:**

To deepen the story, this section briefly discusses the cultural and historical components of fasting. Whether ingrained in religious rites or traditional traditions, knowing the historical backdrop highlights the timelessness of the notion of meal timing. This investigation underscores the premise that the impact of when we eat goes beyond present-day dieting fads.

**Setting the Stage for Personal Transformation:**

As the chapter concludes, it expertly sets the scenario for personal growth. It underlines that intermittent fasting is not a rigorous regimen but a purposeful and empowered lifestyle choice. Readers are advised to regard it as a chance to harness the body's inherent cycles, unleashing the potential for maximum health and comprehensive well-being.

In "Fasting Unveiled," readers begin a deep investigation of the transforming possibilities inherent in the scheduling of meals. This detailed explanation strives to present minute information, guaranteeing a clear knowledge of the vital function that meal timing plays in the tapestry of intermittent fasting.

# Understanding the Impact of Meal Timing on Weight Loss and Health

Meal time is a complicated component of our everyday lives that exceeds the mere act of nutrition, impacting weight control and general well-being. This in-depth examination dives into the subtle link between the timing of meals, weight reduction, and holistic health, shining light on the physiological nuances that underline the significance of when we eat.

## Chronobiology and Circadian Rhythms:

The cornerstone of grasping meal time resides in the field of chronobiology, a study examining our body's internal clock. Circadian rhythms, the natural cycles governing biological functions, play a key role. This section closely investigates how coordinating meal intake with these circadian cycles increases metabolic efficiency. From the peak of digestion throughout the day to overnight repair processes, knowing chronobiology gives insights into why meal timing matters.

**Impact on Metabolism and Insulin Sensitivity:**

Meal time has a tremendous impact on metabolism, altering how our bodies consume and use nutrients. Delving further into this influence exposes the important relationship between meal time and insulin sensitivity. Strategically planned meals help control blood sugar levels, lowering the danger of insulin resistance—an important element not just in weight management but also in the prevention of type 2 diabetes.

**Weight Loss Strategies via Intermittent Fasting:** Transitioning from theory to reality, we study how intermittent fasting leverages smart meal scheduling for optimal weight reduction. Various intermittent fasting patterns, including the common 16:8 strategy and the more intensive OMAD approach, are analyzed. Readers receive practical insights into how changing the timing of eating and fasting intervals promotes fat-burning processes, increases metabolic flexibility, and leads to beneficial changes in body composition. This section attempts to help readers on the route to sustained weight reduction via well-timed meals.

**Hormonal Regulation:**

The delicate dance of hormones—ghrelin and leptin—takes center stage in understanding the influence of meal timing. These hormones, which manage appetite and fullness, are controlled by when we eat. A deep investigation of hormonal control offers readers a full grasp of how mealtime might impact hunger, taking them beyond the typical emphasis on calorie tracking. This understanding helps people to make educated decisions that resonate with their body's natural cycles.

## Beyond Weight Loss: Holistic Health Implications:

While weight reduction is an observable effect, the influence of meal timing goes well beyond appearances. This section discusses the holistic health consequences, spanning improved digestion, higher nutrient absorption, and even better sleep quality. By properly scheduling meals, people may significantly affect their overall well-being, perhaps averting chronic illnesses and contributing to a longer, healthier life. This holistic viewpoint tries to change the emphasis from conventional weight control to a complete approach to health.

## Practical Strategies for Optimal Meal Timing:

Empowering readers with concrete ideas, this part gives practical techniques for adopting healthy meal scheduling into everyday living. From creating regular eating windows to factoring individual circadian cycles, readers are given the skills to handle their unique schedules while enjoying the advantages of well-timed meals. This guarantees that the benefits of meal timing become not simply a theoretical notion but a real and sustainable component of one's lifestyle, boosting both short-term and long-term health improvements.

In this research, we've analyzed the deep web of links between meal time, weight reduction, and holistic health. This article intends to offer readers a thorough awareness of the subtle interaction between when we eat and our physical well-being, enabling them to regard meal time as a strategic component in the quest for optimum health.

# Exploring Different Fasting Regimes and Their Scientific Basis

Fasting is a dynamic domain spanning many regimens, each precisely structured to respond to individual tastes and health aims. In this part, we shall dig into the scientific foundations that support various fasting techniques, providing readers with a full grasp of the physiological subtleties that characterize each program.

## 1. Eating Windows:

The notion of eating windows centers on circadian rhythms and metabolic efficiency. By following a defined timetable for eating, such as the popular 16:8 or 19:5 ratios, people synchronize their meals with the body's natural internal clock. Scientifically, this technique not only manages calorie intake but also guarantees that metabolic functions, including insulin sensitivity and fat utilization, perform properly during the prescribed meal hours.

## 2. OMAD (One Meal a Day):

OMAD provides a more streamlined strategy focused on a single daily meal. Beyond basic calorie restriction, the scientific explanation here dives into the domain of autophagy. Extended fasting periods linked with OMAD induce cellular repair processes, facilitating the elimination of damaged cellular components. This not only assists in the effective functioning of cells but also coincides with hypotheses stating that periodic cellular renewal adds to overall lifespan.

## 3. Up-and-Down-Day Fasting:

The alternating pattern of normal eating days and restricted-calorie or fasting days, indicated by ratios like 5:2, gives a cyclical aspect to fasting. Scientifically, this technique undermines homeostasis, preventing the body from responding to a regular calorie intake. The oscillation between "up days" and "down days" encourages ongoing fat use and metabolic flexibility, giving a varied technique for weight control.

## 4. Extended Fasting:

Extended fasting entails lengthy durations without meals, surpassing 24 hours and frequently reaching several days. The scientific underpinning of this method consists of establishing advanced stages of autophagy and ketosis. Depleting glycogen levels during protracted fasting pushes the body into a condition where it depends on fat storage for energy. While requiring careful thought, protracted fasting may lead to metabolic adaptation and substantial cellular advantages beyond what shorter fasting periods give.

## 5. Hybrid Approaches:

Recognizing the diversity of tastes and aims, some people utilize hybrid fasting practices. By integrating parts from several regimens, people retain a flexible approach that minimizes monotony and continually pushes the metabolism. The scientific logic here is in avoiding adaptation to a particular fasting pattern, preserving continued metabolic reactivity, and averting plateaus in progress.

## Navigating Individualization:

The scientific foundation for the success of various fasting programs is intricately related to individual aspects such as metabolism, lifestyle, and health objectives. Understanding one's individual physiology is crucial for creating a fasting approach that corresponds with specific demands. This individualized approach not only promotes adherence but also optimizes the potential advantages of fasting, realizing that what works effectively for one person may vary for another.

In this part, we addressed the scientific basis of diverse fasting regimens and underlined the delicate interaction between fasting methods and physiological responses. The adaptability of fasting emerges as a strong tool, enabling people to pick a method that resonates ideally with their specific biology and health aspirations.

# The Significance of Timing Meals for Overall Health

Meal timing is not only a ritual; it is a key feature delicately woven into the fabric of our general health. The purpose of this part is to dig even further into the complex relevance of when we eat, revealing the various physiological mechanisms that emphasize the tremendous influence of well-timed meals on overall well-being.

## 1. Circadian Rhythms and Metabolic Synchrony:

Circadian rhythms, frequently referred to as the body's internal clock, coordinate the ebb and flow of biological activities throughout a 24-hour period. Aligning food intake with these natural patterns increases metabolic synchronization. This synchronization increases the efficiency with which the body processes foods, increasing digestion and nutrient absorption. Eating in sync with circadian cycles not only benefits metabolic health but also improves energy use, helping to a balanced and responsive metabolism.

**2. Blood Sugar Regulation and Insulin Sensitivity:**

The timing of meals has a critical role in blood sugar management, directly altering the body's reaction to insulin. Consistent meal time leads to steady blood sugar levels, lowering the risk of insulin resistance. This, in turn, plays a vital role in avoiding type 2 diabetes and developing metabolic resilience. The deliberate alignment of meals with circadian cycles guarantees that the body's insulin response is properly calibrated, promoting long-term metabolic health and lowering the possibility of blood sugar-related disorders.

**3. Hormonal Balance and Appetite Regulation:**

The delicate dance of hunger and satiety hormones, ghrelin and leptin, is dramatically impacted by meal time. Establishing a regular meal plan helps control these hormones, supporting a balanced appetite. This hormonal homeostasis not only benefits in weight control but also creates a healthy connection with food. By honoring the body's natural rhythm, people may negotiate cravings more successfully, make conscious food choices, and create a sustainable attitude toward eating.

## 4. Nutrient Absorption and Digestive Efficiency:

The timing of meals directly affects the efficiency of nutrient absorption. Consuming meals at suitable intervals ensures that the body can absorb critical vitamins and minerals adequately. This has far-reaching ramifications for immunological function, cognitive health, and the general maintenance of key biological systems. Well-timed meals contribute to the body's capacity to obtain maximum nutritional content from the foods ingested, boosting general well-being and vigor.

## 5. Sleep Quality and Chrono-Nutrition:

The impact of meal time extends into the field of sleep quality via the idea of chrono-nutrition.

Late-night eating disturbs circadian rhythms, possibly affecting the body's normal sleep-wake cycle. Understanding the connection between meal timing and circadian rhythms highlights the need to conclude meals well before sleep. This not only assists in improving sleep quality but also leads to greater mental and physical well-being, creating a holistic approach to health that covers both waking and sleeping hours.

## 6. Prevention of Chronic Diseases:

Consistency in well-timed meals appears as a proactive approach against chronic illnesses. Scientific data shows that adopting healthy eating behaviors, including mindful meal scheduling, is connected with a lower risk of illnesses such as heart disease, metabolic syndrome, and particular malignancies. By incorporating well-timed meals into their lifestyle, people actively contribute to their long-term health, developing a solid defense against prospective health difficulties and fostering a proactive approach to disease.

## 7. Psychological Well-being and Routine:

The psychological benefit of well-timed meals goes beyond the physical world. Establishing a regular eating schedule delivers a feeling of structure and predictability, decreasing stress and encouraging mental well-being. A balanced and regular eating schedule not only develops a pleasant connection with food but also adds to emotional resiliency. By adopting mindful meal scheduling into their routine, people create a holistic approach to mental health and psychological well-being, understanding the interrelated nature of physical and mental well-being.

In conclusion, the relevance of timing meals for overall health comprises a complex tapestry of physiological and psychological subtleties. There's a need for attention to the interrelated nature of meal timing with metabolic processes, hormonal balance, food absorption, sleep quality, illness prevention, and psychological well-being. By embracing and emphasizing the strategic timing of meals, people engage on a path toward holistic health, realizing the significant influence that well-timed eating can have on their entire well-being.

# The Role of Fasting in Cultures (e.g., Ramadan)

Fasting, as a cultural phenomenon, stretches much beyond basic abstinence from eating; it weaves a complex tapestry of customs, spiritual depth, social connection, and everlasting wisdom. Examining the importance of fasting in civilizations, with a concentration on Ramadan in Islam, gives a nuanced understanding of how this practice transcends the confines of nutrition to become a cultural landmark.

## 1. Cultural Significance of Fasting:

In many cultures, fasting is profoundly embedded with historical origins, religious beliefs, and a feeling of social identity. Ramadan, celebrated by Muslims globally, serves as a poignant example. Beyond the physical act of fasting, this month functions as a cultural festival, remembering the era when the Quran was revealed. Fasting during Ramadan becomes a shared cultural experience that develops relationships throughout the community, building a collective identity anchored in religion and tradition.

## 2. Spiritual Dimensions of Fasting:

While the physiological advantages of fasting are established, its spiritual components, particularly in cultural settings, provide layers of deep significance.

Ramadan symbolizes this, delivering a spiritual journey defined by self-discipline, meditation, and heightened devotion. Fasting becomes more than a food discipline; it changes into a spiritual activity, prompting people to dive deep, cleanse their spirits, and enhance their relationship with the divine. The act of fasting from eating becomes a channel for spiritual development and attentiveness.

## 3. Communal Aspects of Fasting:

Fasting in civilizations typically goes beyond an individual desire to incorporate social rituals and shared experiences. Ramadan symbolizes this social component, as families and communities join together to break their fasts, share meals, and participate in collective prayers. This social component fosters a feeling of oneness, empathy, and mutual support. It promotes the concept that fasting is not merely a personal undertaking but a shared display of cultural and social identity.

## 4. Rituals & Traditions:

Within the sphere of fasting in civilizations, rituals and customs play a key role. In Ramadan, rituals like the pre-dawn meal (suhoor) and the evening meal to break the fast (iftar) become cultural marks, punctuating each fasting day. These rituals transcend beyond food; they become shared times of delight, meditation, and celebration. Through these traditions, fasting in cultures becomes a dynamic manifestation of cultural heritage, handed down through generations.

**5. Fasting as a Cultural Teacher:**

Beyond its local cultural and religious settings, fasting functions as a universal teacher conveying lessons of discipline, gratitude, and resilience. Across numerous cultures, people deliberately withdraw from worldly luxuries during fasting, cultivating an appreciation for prosperity, empathy for those facing misfortune, and a mentality of thankfulness. Fasting, as a cultural teacher, gives universal insights into the human experience, transcending cultural barriers.

**6. Adaptation to Modern Lifestyles:**

Fasting across cultures displays flexibility to new living while keeping its essential character. In a worldwide environment, people may follow ancient fasting traditions while facing current problems. This adaptation underlines the dynamic character of cultural practices, illustrating how fasting continues to be a relevant and significant element of cultural identity in the face of altering socioeconomic systems.

In conclusion, the function of fasting in societies, demonstrated by rituals like Ramadan, emerges as a diverse cultural phenomenon. It intertwines with history, spirituality, community life, elaborate rites, and eternal teachings. Fasting becomes a cultural light, linking people to their past, spirituality, and the collective knowledge buried in cultural traditions.

# Chapter 2

# Fasting vs. Dieting: The Weight Loss Battle

In the constant quest for successful weight reduction solutions, the contrast between fasting and standard diets becomes a battlefield of methodology. This chapter goes on a full examination, exploring the various processes that set fasting distinct from traditional diets and positioning it as a formidable challenger in the weight reduction field.

## 1. Decoding Weight Loss Mechanisms:

At the foundation of the fasting-dieting duality is a fundamental difference in how they affect the body's systems for losing extra weight. Traditional diets largely depend on calorie restriction, but fasting offers a novel dimension by changing the time of meal consumption. Unraveling the complicated interaction of metabolism, insulin response, and fat utilization lays the basis for understanding how different techniques affect weight reduction results.

## 2. Insulin Sensitivity and Fat Utilization:

A key divergence occurs in the field of insulin sensitivity. Fasting, particularly intermittent fasting, appears to be a strong ally in increasing insulin sensitivity. By establishing times of dietary abstention, fasting mitigates insulin resistance, allowing the body to effectively use stored fat for energy. This is in contrast to typical diets, which, although lowering calorie consumption, may not have the same favorable influence on insulin sensitivity.

## 3. Hormonal Responses:

The weight reduction war extends into the arena of hormonal reactions, where fasting reveals its ability to orchestrate beneficial hormonal surges. Intermittent fasting, for instance, produces a rise in norepinephrine and human growth hormone, both crucial in promoting fat mobilization and speeding metabolism. These hormonal fluctuations produce an environment favorable to effective fat-burning, separating fasting from the typical techniques of dieting.

**4. Metabolic Adaptation and Plateau Avoidance:**

Traditional diets generally battle with the difficulty of metabolic adaptation, when the body responds to decreased calorie intake by slowing down metabolism. Fasting presents purposeful variability with its intermittent nature, minimizing this adaptation problem. By integrating times of normal eating, fasting prevents the body from settling into a chronic state of lowered metabolism, enabling a proactive technique to overcome plateaus in the weight reduction path.

## 5. Psychological Impact and Sustained Adherence:

Beyond physiological differences, the psychological effect of fasting vs dieting arises as a significant concern. Fasting, with its set eating windows and times of abstinence, may appeal better to persons seeking order and simplicity. The lack of continual calorie tracking and tight dietary limitations create a sustainable approach, perhaps leading to better adherence compared to the often-restrictive character of conventional diets.

## 6. Long-Term Weight Maintenance:

The weight reduction fight goes beyond dropping pounds to the domain of long-term weight management. Fasting, with its capacity to retain lean muscle mass and enhance fat use, promotes itself as a competitor for prolonged weight control. Traditional diets, which may accidentally contribute to muscle loss and metabolic slowness, confront obstacles in assuring durable weight control.

## 7. Scientific Rationale and Evidence:

Anchoring the discussion of fasting vs dieting is a rigorous assessment of the scientific reasoning supporting each technique. Fasting, especially intermittent fasting, relies on a firm foundation of studies emphasizing its good impacts on metabolic health, insulin control, and fat oxidation. This scientific underpinning leads to the increased acknowledgment of fasting as a valid and evidence-based technique for weight reduction.

In short, Chapter 2 goes a detailed voyage into the subtle dynamics of the weight reduction fight, presenting an in-depth review of the opposing techniques of fasting and dieting. By unraveling the physiological, hormonal, and psychological elements, this chapter offers people a nuanced knowledge to traverse the complicated terrain of weight reduction techniques, supporting informed decision-making on their path toward reaching and maintaining a healthy weight.

# Why Fasting Prevails Over Traditional Diets for Weight Loss

In the unceasing quest for successful weight reduction solutions, the supremacy of fasting over standard diets emerges as a tale replete with scientific rationale and practical benefits. This section digs further into the multifaceted reasons why fasting stands out as an effective and sustainable technique for reducing extra weight, outshining the conventional paradigms of typical dieting.

**1. Metabolic Flexibility and Fat Utilization:**

Fasting advocates the notion of metabolic flexibility, a vital feature contributing to its success in weight reduction. Unlike conventional diets that largely depend on calorie reduction, fasting incorporates times of food abstention. This purposeful fasting and feasting cycle urges the body to adapt to different energy sources, encouraging greater metabolic flexibility. The outcome is enhanced use of stored fat for energy, presenting fasting as a potent accelerator for fat reduction without the difficulties associated with extended calorie restriction.

## 2. Insulin Sensitivity and Hormonal Harmony:

A particular edge of fasting resides in its good influence on insulin sensitivity and hormonal equilibrium. Intermittent fasting, in particular, appears as a strategic strategy to minimize insulin resistance, a typical stumbling block in weight reduction trips. By controlling insulin levels via intermittent fasting cycles, an environment favorable to effective fat mobilization is established. Moreover, the hormonal response induced by fasting, including heightened levels of norepinephrine and human growth hormone, not only boosts metabolism but also enhances the body's capacity to burn fat efficiently.

## 3. Avoidance of Metabolic Adaptation:

Traditional diets generally battle with the difficulty of metabolic adaptation, when the body responds to decreased calorie intake by slowing down metabolism. Fasting deliberately navigates this hurdle by its intermittent nature. By combining times of ordinary eating, fasting reduces the metabolic slowing associated with extended calorie restriction. This dynamic technique provides a proactive way to prevent plateaus in the weight reduction journey, assuring continued progress and outcomes.

## 4. Psychological Resilience and Sustainable Adherence:

The psychological component becomes a crucial reason for favoring fasting over typical diets.

Fasting, characterized by fixed meal windows and planned times of abstinence, offers a disciplined but adjustable method of weight control. This simplicity connects with folks seeking a durable and psychologically robust strategy. The absence of continual calorie tracking and rigorous dietary limitations develops a pleasant connection with food, boosting long-term adherence to the weight-reduction plan and encouraging a healthy perspective toward nutrition.

## 5. Preservation of Lean Muscle Mass:

An often-overlooked component is the retention of lean muscle mass during fasting. Traditional diets, particularly those containing considerable calorie limitations, may lead to unintentional muscle loss with fat reduction. Fasting, however, favors the maintenance of lean muscle mass. This not only aids in developing a toned body but also plays a significant part in maintaining weight reduction over the long run. Preserving muscle mass ensures that the weight lost predominantly includes fat, resulting in a more favorable body composition.

## 6. Enhanced Autophagy and Cellular Health:

Fasting introduces the interesting notion of autophagy, a cellular self-cleaning mechanism with substantial implications for weight reduction and general health. During fasting, the body activates autophagy, a procedure that tears down damaged cells and cellular components. This method goes beyond basic fat loss, actively promoting cellular health and perhaps giving lifespan and well-being advantages. The combination of fasting-induced autophagy with weight reduction underlines the comprehensive influence of fasting on overall health.

## 7. Scientific Validation and Research Support:

The popularity of fasting as a better weight reduction approach receives substantial backing in scientific validation and study. Numerous studies continuously underline the usefulness of intermittent fasting in encouraging weight reduction, enhancing metabolic health, and presenting a sustainable method for long-term weight control. This scientific evidence not only substantiates the claims of fasting proponents but also portrays fasting as more than a fleeting craze. It validates its standing as an evidence-based and dependable technique for reaching weight reduction objectives, creating confidence in those beginning on their weight loss journey.

In summary, the success of fasting over standard diets for weight reduction unfolds as a multidimensional tale, integrating physiological, hormonal, psychological, and scientific components. This section explains why fasting stands as a compelling and sustainable paradigm, redefining the narrative surrounding weight reduction and offering people a strong and evidence-based tool to attain and maintain a healthy body weight.

# Exploring the Unique Mechanisms of Fasting for Fat Loss

In the multifaceted terrain of weight management, fasting stands as a distinctive technique, wielding specific processes that separate it from typical weight reduction treatments. This in-depth examination unravels the subtleties underpinning fasting's effectiveness in fat reduction, diving into the physiological intricacies and providing light on why it defies standard paradigms in the field of weight management.

**1. Metabolic Switch to Fat Utilization:**

Fasting orchestrates a dramatic metabolic change inside the body. During times of fasting, when glucose levels decrease in the absence of food intake, the body shifts from using glucose as its major energy source to depending on stored fat. This metabolic response, known as ketosis, is typified by accelerated lipolysis—the breakdown of fat into fatty acids and glycerol. Unlike traditional diets that largely concentrate on calorie restriction, fasting generates a physiological state where fat becomes a primary and efficient fuel for energy.

## 2. Hormonal Regulation for Optimal Fat Mobilization:

The effectiveness of fasting in encouraging fat reduction is closely connected to its capacity to modulate hormones. Insulin, a hormone that prevents fat breakdown, diminishes during fasting, allowing fat cells to release stored fatty acids. Concurrently, chemicals like norepinephrine and human growth hormone see a spike, stimulating the breakdown of fat for energy. This hormonal interaction highlights the efficacy of fasting in establishing an environment where the body becomes skilled at mobilizing and using its fat stores.

**3. Induction of Ketosis:**

Fasting creates a metabolic state known as ketosis, a process when the body largely depends on ketone bodies obtained from fat breakdown as its major fuel source. This condition, separate from the glucose-dependent metabolism found in conventional diets, promotes fat burning. The metabolic change to ketosis is a crucial component of the prolonged fat loss seen in fasting, as the body becomes adept at turning stored fat into ketones for energy.

## 4. Enhanced Caloric Restriction without the Pitfalls:

While fasting offers an aspect of caloric restriction, it does so without some of the difficulties associated with continuous calorie reduction. Traditional diets often lead to a drop in metabolic rate and the loss of lean muscle mass. Fasting, however, tends to retain lean muscle mass, guaranteeing that the weight lost is largely fat. This preservation not only aids in attaining a toned body but is also vital for preserving fat reduction in the long term.

**5. Autophagy and Cellular Cleansing:**

A distinctive element of fasting is the introduction of autophagy, a cellular self-cleansing mechanism. During fasting, the body recognizes and destroys damaged or defective cellular components. This process helps not just cellular health but also aids fat reduction. The clearance of unproductive cells promotes a more streamlined and efficient cellular environment, generating circumstances favorable to prolonged fat reduction.

**6. Breaking Insulin Resistance:**

Fasting addresses a common obstacle to fat loss—insulin resistance. Regular fasting intervals can reduce insulin resistance by decreasing total insulin levels. Lower insulin levels boost the body's capacity to mobilize and use fat for energy, making fasting a helpful method for persons encountering difficulty in weight reduction owing to insulin-related disorders.

**7. Psychological Impact for Sustainable Adherence:**

Beyond its physiological mechanics, fasting includes a psychological factor that leads to lasting fat reduction. The regular eating windows and planned times of abstention build a good connection with food. This psychological resilience promotes adherence to the fasting regimen, ensuring that patients can continuously follow the protocol—a critical aspect in reaching and sustaining fat reduction objectives over the long run.

In summary, the examination of the specific processes of fasting for fat reduction uncovers a thorough interaction of metabolic, hormonal, and psychological components. Fasting's capacity to create a metabolic flip, control hormones, establish ketosis, promote autophagy, address insulin resistance, and encourage psychological resilience puts it as a complex and powerful treatment for those seeking not just effective but also sustained fat reduction.

# Impact of Fasting on Insulin Levels and Fat Burning

Fasting, especially intermittent fasting, has a dramatic impact on insulin levels and the delicate process of fat burning inside the body. Understanding this impact uncovers critical processes that contribute to the success of fasting as a strategy for weight control and general metabolic health.

## 1. Regulation of Insulin Levels:

Insulin, a hormone generated by the pancreas, plays a crucial function in glucose metabolism. Its principal purpose is to enhance the absorption of glucose into cells, where it may be utilized for energy or stored as glycogen. However, chronic increased insulin levels, frequently linked with continuous eating practices, may lead to insulin resistance—a condition where cells become less sensitive to insulin signals, resulting in weight gain and metabolic disorders.

Fasting adds a vital feature of insulin control. During fasting periods, particularly in intermittent fasting regimens, the body experiences a considerable drop in insulin production. This decrease assists in disrupting the loop of continuous insulin exposure, encouraging greater insulin sensitivity over time. Enhanced insulin sensitivity is linked with more efficient glucose management, lower risk of type 2 diabetes, and, significantly, a favorable environment for fat burning.

**2. Fat Burning in the Absence of Insulin:**

Insulin and fat burning have an inverse connection. When insulin levels are high, the body prioritizes glucose as its major energy source and slows the breakdown of fat for fuel. Conversely, during fasting, times when insulin is low, the body experiences a metabolic change. In the absence of insulin signaling, cells become more sensitive to using stored fat as an energy source.

Intermittent fasting, with its alternating cycles of eating and fasting, enables the body to enter stages when insulin is decreased. This offers windows of opportunity for efficient fat burning. As the body dips into its fat reserves for energy, people engaging in intermittent fasting frequently see a considerable drop in body fat percentage over time.

**3. Enhanced Lipolysis and Fat Mobilization:**

Fasting accelerates a process known as lipolysis when stored fat is broken down into fatty acids and glycerol. This process is assisted by hormones such as norepinephrine, which become more prominent during fasting times. Norepinephrine, along with other hormones, including human growth hormone, actively stimulates the mobilization of fat from adipose tissue.

The combination of lower insulin levels and enhanced lipolysis generates an environment favorable to effective fat mobilization. Fasting, then, not only permits the body to use existing fat reserves for energy but also facilitates the breakdown of triglycerides into fatty acids—a vital stage in the fat-burning process.

## 4. Mitigation of Metabolic Syndrome:

Metabolic syndrome, defined by a cluster of diseases including high blood pressure, excessive blood sugar, extra belly fat, and abnormal cholesterol levels, is intimately connected to insulin resistance. Fasting, via its influence on insulin levels, tackles one of the core reasons for metabolic syndrome.

By improving insulin sensitivity and decreasing insulin resistance, fasting aids in the prevention and treatment of metabolic syndrome. The decrease in belly fat, commonly noted with fasting-induced fat burning, further contributes to improving overall metabolic health and lowering the risk of related problems.

**5. Long-Term Benefits for Weight Management:**

The influence of fasting on insulin levels and fat burning persists beyond immediate effects. Long-term adherence to intermittent fasting has been linked with durable gains in insulin sensitivity, even during feeding periods. This prolonged advantage emphasizes the promise of fasting not just as a short-term weight control method but as a lifestyle approach that favorably improves metabolic health over the long run.

In summary, the influence of fasting on insulin levels and fat burning is a dynamic interaction that addresses essential elements of metabolic health. By controlling insulin, increasing efficient fat mobilization, and alleviating metabolic syndrome, fasting emerges as a strategic and sustainable option for those seeking successful weight management and better overall health.

# Understanding How Fasting Affects Hunger Hormones and Metabolism

Fasting, especially intermittent fasting, orchestrates a complicated dance involving hunger hormones and metabolic processes inside the body. This delicate interaction not only determines how we perceive hunger but also has major consequences on metabolism, adding to the effectiveness of fasting as a weight control method and enhancing overall metabolic health.

## 1. Regulation of Ghrelin: The Hunger Hormone:

Ghrelin, frequently referred to as the "hunger hormone," is a critical factor in human experiences of hunger. Produced predominantly in the stomach, ghrelin tells the brain to boost hunger and the urge to eat. During fasting periods, particularly in the beginning stages, ghrelin levels tend to rise. This rise in ghrelin acts as a physiological reaction, indicating the body's anticipation of eating.

However, the intriguing feature of fasting comes in its potential to change the ghrelin response over time. With a continued commitment to intermittent fasting, people frequently undergo a recalibration of ghrelin levels. This recalibration translates into a more controlled and predictable hunger pattern, leading to improved appetite control and fewer impulsive eating.

## 2. Leptin: The Satiety Hormone:

Leptin, commonly nicknamed the "satiety hormone," functions in opposition to ghrelin. Produced by fat cells, leptin signals to the brain when the body has eaten enough to eat, fostering a sensation of fullness and contentment. Traditional diets, particularly those stressing calorie restriction, may affect leptin levels, leading to diminished satiety signals and increased sensations of hunger. Intermittent fasting, however, seems to have a favorable influence on leptin sensitivity. By producing separate cycles of eating and fasting, the body becomes more responsive to leptin signals. This heightened sensitivity leads to enhanced appetite management, making it simpler for people to perceive and react to actual hunger signals while also boosting the overall satiety sensation during eating windows.

## 3. Metabolic Adaptations: Fasting and Insulin Sensitivity:

Beyond the area of hunger hormones, fasting has a substantial effect on metabolic adaptations, notably in connection to insulin sensitivity. Insulin, a hormone necessary for glucose homeostasis, is closely tied to both hunger and metabolism. Continuous exposure to elevated insulin levels, frequently found in traditional eating habits, may develop into insulin resistance, affecting metabolic health and leading to weight gain.

Fasting produces a fundamental change in insulin dynamics. During fasting times, insulin levels decline, enabling the body to become more sensitive to its effects. This higher insulin sensitivity boosts the body's capacity to properly utilize glucose for energy, reducing excessive accumulation of fat. The metabolic adaptations created by fasting contribute not just to efficient weight control but also to overall metabolic health.

## 4. Ketosis and Appetite Suppression:

Intermittent fasting, particularly when prolonged over longer durations, sometimes generates a condition of ketosis. Ketosis is defined by the usage of ketone bodies, produced from fat breakdown, as a major energy source. This metabolic state goes hand-in-hand with hunger suppression.

Ketone bodies have an appetite-suppressing impact, altering the areas of the brain responsible for controlling hunger. As the body goes into ketosis during fasting, people commonly report a lower feeling of hunger, making it simpler to stick to fasting protocols and experience extended periods of reduced calorie intake.

## 5. Enhanced Fat Oxidation and Weight Loss:

Fasting promotes improved fat oxidation, a process where the body effectively uses stored fat for energy. This goes beyond the mere idea of calorie restriction since fasting particularly targets fat storage. The increased dependence on fat for fuel leads to persistent weight reduction, with a large amount of the lost weight deriving from stored fat rather than lean muscle mass.

The connection between fasting, hunger hormones, and metabolism provides a synergistic impact that goes beyond basic weight control. It generates a metabolic milieu favorable to long-term health advantages, including enhanced insulin sensitivity, better appetite management, and efficient fat utilization.

In conclusion, knowing how fasting impacts hunger hormones and metabolism gives useful insights into the varied advantages of intermittent fasting. By regulating ghrelin and leptin, improving insulin sensitivity, inducing ketosis, and encouraging fat oxidation, fasting appears not just as a potent tool for weight control but as a holistic approach supporting total metabolic well-being.

# Chapter 3

# The Expansive Benefits of Fasting

Fasting, generally considered a food method, emerges as a transforming lifestyle strategy with a range of advantages that delicately weave into the fabric of human health and lifespan. This chapter goes into a deep investigation of the various benefits given by intermittent fasting, providing light on the subtle processes that drive its influence on many areas of physical and mental well-being.

**1. Autophagy: Cellular Regeneration and Repair:**

Autophagy, the cellular self-cleaning mechanism engaged during fasting, digs into the subtleties of cellular health. This procedure goes beyond normal maintenance; it's a thorough sorting mechanism that finds and disposes of damaged cellular components.

The consequences extend beyond the available possible lifespan since the elimination of damaged parts supports a cellular milieu favorable to optimum functioning and resistance against age-related deterioration.

Autophagy, operating as a biological restoration, has been linked to lowered risks of neurodegenerative illnesses and an overall increase in cellular vitality. The ongoing cycle of repair and rejuvenation begun by autophagy positions fasting as a potent proponent of cellular lifespan.

## 2. Inflammation Reduction and Longevity:

The voyage into fasting's advantages delves into the world of inflammation reduction—a critical aspect in the search for increased health span. Chronic inflammation is linked to different illnesses, from cardiovascular difficulties to autoimmune disorders. Intermittent fasting's power to suppress inflammatory indicators has a dramatic anti-aging impact, possibly lowering the risk of age-related diseases.

In the search for longevity, inhibition of inflammatory pathways appears as a major technique. Fasting, because of its anti-inflammatory action, is a prophylactic intervention against illnesses related to chronic inflammation. This anti-aging potential frames fasting as a comprehensive strategy for achieving a longer and healthier life.

## 3. Enhanced Brain Function and Cognitive Health:

The story of fasting transcends the bodily to incorporate cognitive well-being. As the body reaches a state of ketosis during fasting, the brain obtains a regular and efficient energy source, encouraging mental clarity and cognitive performance. Beyond basic energy availability, fasting begins the creation of brain-derived neurotrophic factor (BDNF), a neuroprotective ingredient that promotes the development and maintenance of neurons.

Fasting's effect on sustaining cognitive function extends to possible protection against neurodegenerative disorders. The complicated interaction between ketosis and neurotrophic factors frames fasting as a tempting method for preserving cognitive vibrancy and perhaps postponing the start of age-related cognitive decline.

**4. Blood Sugar Regulation and Diabetes Prevention:**

At the root of metabolic health lies the management of blood sugar levels—a realm where intermittent fasting reveals its brilliance. By improving insulin sensitivity and decreasing insulin resistance, fasting becomes a proactive intervention in the prevention and control of type 2 diabetes. The rigorous engineering of insulin dynamics puts fasting as a cornerstone in promoting metabolic resilience.

Stabilized blood sugar levels not only help with diabetes prevention but also play a crucial role in sustaining energy levels and overall metabolic homeostasis. Fasting's entire influence on blood sugar management surpasses immediate health advantages, setting the framework for long-term metabolic well-being.

## 5. Heart health and disease prevention:

The canvas of fasting's advantages broadens to include the delicate tapestry of cardiovascular health. Beyond its acknowledged function in weight control, intermittent fasting displays a substantial effect on cardiovascular risk factors. The lowering of blood pressure, improvement in cholesterol profiles, and decrease in triglyceride levels all contribute to a heart-healthy environment.

As a comprehensive approach to heart health, fasting not only treats urgent difficulties but also functions as a prophylactic precaution against cardiovascular illnesses. The potential lifespan linked to a healthy circulatory system magnifies the influence of fasting on general well-being.

## 6. Cancer Prevention and Supportive Therapy:

While research on fasting's influence on cancer prevention is an ongoing domain, new data indicates its possible importance. Fasting's multi-faceted effect, from inflammation reduction to better immune function and cellular repair, corresponds with techniques in cancer prevention and supportive treatment.

The caveat resides in the continuing study, underscoring the necessity for a comprehensive understanding of fasting's consequences in the complex terrain of cancer. As research emerges, fasting may emerge as a supporting aspect in the prevention and treatment of some malignancies, adding another dimension to its wide advantages.

## 7. Improved Gut Health and Microbiome Balance:

Venturing into the depths of digestive well-being, intermittent fasting helps to maintain the delicate balance of the gut flora. A healthy and diversified microbial population inside the digestive tract is related to better digestion, greater nutritional absorption, and a lower risk of gastrointestinal disorders.

Fasting's favorable effect on gut health stretches beyond immediate digestive advantages, producing an environment that promotes general well-being. The symbiotic interaction between fasting and the gut flora adds a degree of complexity to its entire influence on the body.

## 8. Psychological Well-Being and Mindful Eating:

In the field of psychological well-being, fasting provides a distinct dimension to our connection with food. Structured eating windows and purposeful times of abstention foster awareness of eating behaviors. This purposeful and aware approach to food intake leads to lower stress, greater mental resilience, and a positive attitude toward one's relationship with nutrition.

# Beyond Weight Loss: Unveiling Extensive Health Benefits of Fasting

While fasting has earned a reputation as an effective weight management approach, its profound influence goes well beyond dropping pounds. This investigation exposes the wide health advantages that intermittent fasting provides, breaking the usual confines of dieting and providing a comprehensive approach to well-being.

**1. Metabolic Flexibility and Energy Efficiency:**

Intermittent fasting acts as a catalyst for metabolic flexibility, a condition when the body fluidly shifts between burning glucose and dipping it into stored fat for energy. This metabolic flexibility not only assists in weight control but also promotes overall energy efficiency. Fasting prepares the body to be resourceful, guaranteeing a consistent flow of energy even during situations of food shortage.

This metabolic adaptability adds to prolonged vigor and may play a role in avoiding energy-related diseases, giving a dynamic perspective on the larger health advantages connected with fasting.

**2. Cellular Resilience and Longevity:**

Fasting increases cellular stress response pathways, pushing cells to build their defenses and adapt to harsh environments. This cellular resilience, created by intermittent fasting, is connected to an improved lifespan. The periodic stresses imposed by fasting activate cellular repair processes, minimizing the risk of age-related illnesses and fostering a more resilient cellular environment.

Beyond the immediate objective of weight reduction, fasting appears as a technique for cellular renewal, perhaps opening the path for a longer and healthier life.

## 3. Hormonal Harmony and Endocrine Health:

The fasting paradigm orchestrates a complex balance in hormone regulation, regulating major players such as insulin, ghrelin, and leptin. Insulin sensitivity increases, lowering the likelihood of insulin resistance and type 2 diabetes. Ghrelin, the hunger hormone, undergoes modification, leading to improved appetite control. Simultaneously, leptin, which is responsible for signaling fullness, becomes more effective.

This hormonal equilibrium not only benefits weight control but also tackles underlying metabolic abnormalities, positioning fasting as a complete approach to endocrine health.

## 4. Enhanced Immune Function:

Fasting has been associated with increases in immunological function, increasing the body's defensive systems against infections and illnesses. During fasting times, the immune system undertakes a renewing process, cleaning away old or damaged cells and creating space for new, more effective ones. This immune boost offers a layer of protection against common diseases and may lead to a lower risk of chronic inflammatory problems.

Beyond the cosmetic objective of weight reduction, fasting appears as a proactive method for reinforcing the body's inherent defense.

## 5. Cognitive Clarity and Brain Health:

The cognitive advantages of intermittent fasting extend beyond weight-related results. Fasting causes a condition of ketosis when the brain utilizes ketones as an alternate energy source. This metabolic change is related to heightened cognitive clarity, increased attention, and perhaps a decreased risk of neurodegenerative illnesses.

As a comprehensive approach to brain health, fasting not only assists in weight control but also fosters cognitive well-being, delivering a compelling incentive for individuals seeking mental sharpness and resilience.

## 6. Cardiovascular Resilience:

The cardiovascular system reaps advantages beyond weight-related reductions with intermittent fasting. Fasting relates to lower blood pressure, better lipid profiles, and increased vascular health. These cardiovascular advantages position fasting as a holistic approach to heart resilience, possibly decreasing the risk of cardiovascular illnesses.

In essence, fasting becomes more than a tool for weight control—it becomes a proactive approach for maintaining a robust and resilient cardiovascular system.

## 7. Anti-Inflammatory Effects:

Chronic inflammation is a common denominator in different health concerns, from arthritis to heart disease. Intermittent fasting has powerful anti-inflammatory benefits by lowering inflammatory markers. This anti-inflammatory activity not only assists with weight-related difficulties but also targets the underlying inflammation linked to various chronic conditions. Fasting emerges as a comprehensive anti-inflammatory therapy, delivering advantages that reach far beyond the scale and establishing a systemic milieu favorable to general health.

## 8. Cellular Recycling and Detoxification:

Autophagy, the cellular recycling mechanism engaged during fasting, plays a crucial function in detoxifying the body. It recognizes and eliminates damaged cellular components, enhancing cellular cleanliness and efficiency. This cellular detoxification, beyond its consequences for weight reduction, adds to a better internal environment, possibly lowering the risk of cellular malfunction and associated disorders.

In summary, the health advantages of intermittent fasting transcend the single emphasis on weight reduction. From metabolic flexibility to cellular resilience, hormonal balance, immunological enhancement, cognitive well-being, cardiovascular resilience, anti-inflammatory benefits, and cellular cleansing, fasting emerges as a complete approach for enhancing holistic health and longevity.

# Fasting's Role in Reducing Insulin and Preventing Type 2 Diabetes: A Deeper Dive

The delicate link between intermittent fasting, insulin dynamics, and the prevention of type 2 diabetes emerges as a sophisticated inquiry into the physiological principles that underlie metabolic health.

**1. Insulin Sensitivity Enhancement:**

Insulin sensitivity, the efficiency with which cells react to insulin's regulatory signals, is at the foundation of diabetes prevention. Intermittent fasting functions as a catalyst in this situation, improving insulin sensitivity via several methods. During fasting periods, the body's cells endure a lower inflow of nutrients, pushing them to become more sensitive to insulin. This heightened sensitivity enables the effective absorption of glucose, lowering the stress on the insulin-producing mechanism.

The subtle dance of insulin sensitivity enhancement sets the setting for a balanced metabolic environment, critical for resisting the establishment of insulin resistance and, ultimately, diabetes.

## 2. Mitigation of Insulin Resistance:

Insulin resistance, a crucial element in the path toward type 2 diabetes, includes cells opposing insulin's efforts to control blood sugar. Intermittent fasting intervenes in this process by disrupting the loop of continuous nutrient exposure. Fasting times give cells a break, enabling them to reset and recover reactivity to insulin.

This reduction of insulin resistance becomes a significant tactic, interrupting the trajectory toward diabetes by treating one of its fundamental antecedents.

### 3. Blood Sugar Regulation:

The orchestration of blood sugar levels becomes a finely tuned symphony under the influence of intermittent fasting. During fasting periods, the dependence on stored glucose induces a regulated and progressive release into the circulation. This coordinated regulation of blood sugar levels fits with the body's natural ebb and flow, preventing the sudden spikes and falls associated with diabete

The rhythmic modulation of blood sugar emerges as a preventative approach, minimizing the burden on insulin and supporting glucose homeostasis.

## 4. Beta-Cell Function Preservation:

Beta cells, snuggled inside the pancreas, have the task of insulin synthesis. Prolonged periods of high insulin demand, commonly induced by frequent meals, may strain and impair these important cells. Intermittent fasting offers times of decreased insulin production, enabling beta cells to recuperate and retain their function.

The maintenance of beta-cell function becomes a proactive approach, shielding against the beta-cell malfunction that precedes the development of type 2 diabetes.

## 5. Inflammatory Control and Diabetes Prevention:

Chronic inflammation is both a result and a factor in insulin resistance and diabetes. Intermittent fasting's anti-inflammatory actions play a vital role in developing an internal milieu resistant to the inflammatory processes linked with diabetes. By limiting inflammation, fasting provides a foundation for strong metabolic health.

This combined action—addressing inflammation and fine-tuning insulin dynamics—positions fasting as a complete and systemic strategy for avoiding type 2 diabetes.

**6. Weight Management as a Contributing Factor:**

While not the main emphasis, weight control acts as a vital component of diabetes prevention. Intermittent fasting, through its regulation of insulin and general metabolic improvement, leads to sustained weight management. The decrease in excess body weight creates an extra layer of protection against the numerous dangers connected with type 2 diabetes.

The comprehensive approach of fasting, involving both insulin control and weight management, confirms its effectiveness in the larger context of diabetes prevention.

In summary, the subtle dance between intermittent fasting, insulin sensitivity, and type 2 diabetes prevention includes a symphony of physiological adjustments. From boosting insulin sensitivity and moderating insulin resistance to coordinating blood sugar homeostasis, protecting beta-cell function, regulating inflammation, and helping with weight management, fasting uncovers itself as a complex and proactive method for safeguarding metabolic health.

# Addressing Chronic Inflammation via Fasting: A Deeper Dive.

The war against chronic inflammation takes on a subtle complexity when examined through the lens of intermittent fasting, uncovering a tapestry of interwoven physiological responses that actively strive to prevent the insidious consequences of persistent inflammation.

## 1. Understanding Chronic Inflammation:

Chronic inflammation is a complicated and varied biological response that becomes deleterious when it continues over lengthy durations. Triggered by a range of causes, including poor food choices, stress, and lifestyle factors, chronic inflammation is linked to the genesis and progression of several illnesses. Its subtle, systemic nature makes it a quiet contributor to ailments ranging from cardiovascular problems to metabolic disorders.

## 2. Fasting's Anti-Inflammatory Mechanisms:

Intermittent fasting, as a proactive technique, engages in a complicated tango with the body's inflammatory pathways. Fasting generates a condition of physiological rest during non-eating times, enabling the body to shift its attention from digestion to cellular repair and regeneration. This metabolic recalibration increases autophagy, a process where damaged cellular components are disassembled and recycled, dramatically lowering the inflammatory triggers inside cells.

Moreover, fasting serves as a gatekeeper against the inflow of pro-inflammatory chemicals commonly linked with processed and calorie-dense diets. By limiting dietary intake, fasting curtails the basic ingredients that drive chronic inflammation.

## 3. Hormonal Regulation and Inflammation:

Fasting orchestrates a symphony of hormonal control, where insulin and cortisol take center stage. Insulin sensitivity increases, lowering the risk of inflammation associated with insulin resistance. Simultaneously, cortisol, a hormone integrally connected to stress and inflammation, enjoys a balanced ebb and flow during fasting. This hormonal homeostasis creates an anti-inflammatory environment inside the body.

## 4. Impact on Adipose Tissue and Inflammatory Markers:

Excess adipose tissue, especially visceral fat, becomes a battlefield in the combat against chronic inflammation. Intermittent fasting's focus on metabolic efficiency and weight control directly addresses this adipose storage. By lowering visceral fat, fasting decreases the generation of inflammatory cytokines and markers, interrupting the inflammatory cascade linked with adipose tissue.

## 5. Autophagy and Cellular Cleanliness:

Beyond repair, autophagy initiated by fasting adds to cellular cleanliness—an often-overlooked facet of inflammation regulation. By removing defective cellular components, autophagy inhibits the buildup of inflammatory stimuli, preserving cellular homeostasis and minimizing the possibility of chronic inflammation.


**6. Preventing Inflammatory-Driven Diseases:**

Chronic inflammation acts as a common denominator in the development of many illnesses. Intermittent fasting, with its comprehensive approach, emerges as a strong guardian against inflammatory-driven illnesses. Whether it's atherosclerosis, insulin resistance, or autoimmune illnesses, fasting serves as a proactive defense, interrupting the underlying inflammatory processes.

## 7. Long-Term Inflammatory Resilience:

Consistency in intermittent fasting builds prolonged resistance to chronic inflammation. The periodic nature of fasting limits the continual exposure to inflammatory stimuli, enabling the body to reset and maintain a balanced inflammatory response. This persistent resilience is not only vital for immediate health advantages but also acts as a protective strategy against inflammatory illnesses that can appear over time.

## 8. Collaboration with Other Health Strategies:

Fasting synergizes with alternative health methods, such as a nutrient-dense diet and frequent physical exercise. This partnership develops a comprehensive approach to inflammation treatment, where intermittent fasting functions as a basic pillar in developing resilience and reinforcing the body against the persistent challenges of chronic inflammation.

In essence, the complicated interaction between intermittent fasting and chronic inflammation includes a ballet of physiological changes. From triggering autophagy and hormone control to influencing adipose tissue and avoiding inflammatory-driven disorders, fasting appears as a complete and sophisticated technique. Beyond weight control, it becomes a watchful guardian, aggressively addressing and moderating the quiet inflammatory factors that risk long-term health and well-being.

# Exploring the Link Between Fasting and Longevity: A Comprehensive Insight

Embarking on a thorough investigation of the relationship between intermittent fasting and longevity leads us on a trip through the various physiological systems that emphasize the possibility of a longer, healthier life. Let's look further into each part of this interesting relationship.

## 1. Cellular Rejuvenation by Autophagy:

At the crux of fasting's influence on lifespan lies the phenomenon of autophagy. This sophisticated cellular process is analogous to cellular spring-cleaning, when the body launches a self-cleansing mechanism, breaking down and recycling damaged or defective cellular components. The coordinated dance of autophagy not only helps to enhance cellular health and functioning but also coincides with the belief that a cleaner, more efficient cellular environment may pave the way for a longer lifespan. Research shows that the frequent activation of autophagy by intermittent fasting may play a vital role in slowing down the aging process at the cellular level.

**2. Mitigation of Oxidative Stress:**

Aging is commonly accompanied by oxidative stress, a process caused by an imbalance between free radicals and the body's capacity to neutralize them using antioxidants. Intermittent fasting appears as a major mitigating mechanism against oxidative stress. By increasing the body's antioxidant defenses, fasting functions as a buffer against the cellular damage and wear and tear associated with aging. This decrease in oxidative stress is not only a cosmetic upgrade; it offers the possibility of prolonging overall longevity by protecting the integrity of critical cellular components.

**3. Inflammation Control and Age-Related Diseases:**

Chronic inflammation, a typical companion to the aging process, is a promoter of many age-related disorders. Fasting's significant anti-inflammatory benefits come forward as a prophylactic approach. By regulating chronic inflammation, intermittent fasting tackles a basic cause of several illnesses connected with aging, ranging from cardiovascular difficulties to neurological disorders. The sophisticated regulation of inflammatory reactions frames fasting as a comprehensive approach for boosting long-term health and lifespan.

## 4. Enhancement of Cellular Repair Processes:

Beyond the boundaries of autophagy, fasting extends its effect to other key cellular repair processes, including DNA repair. The periodic stress imposed by fasting activates cellular repair mechanisms, boosting resistance against the accumulation of genetic defects associated with aging. By actively participating in DNA repair, intermittent fasting aids in preserving genetic integrity, a cornerstone for good aging and perhaps an extended lifetime.

**5. Impact on Insulin Sensitivity and Metabolic Health:**

Insulin resistance, a characteristic of the aging process, is closely connected to metabolic health and lifespan. Intermittent fasting's favorable influence on insulin sensitivity plays a significant role in this narrative. The precise balance maintained via fasting helps manage blood sugar levels, minimizing the risk of age-related metabolic diseases such as type 2 diabetes. By maintaining adequate insulin function, intermittent fasting not only improves metabolic health but also coincides with the hypothesis that regulating these essential pathways may lead to a longer lifetime.

## 6. Promotion of Healthy Weight Management:

While not the primary determinant, keeping a healthy weight is a vital aspect of lifespan. Intermittent fasting, with its multidimensional approach to weight control, makes a substantial contribution to a healthy body composition. The decrease in excess body weight, especially visceral fat, is connected with a reduced risk of age-related disorders. Fasting's effect on healthy weight dynamics makes it a real component in enhancing overall lifespan.

## 7. Sirtuins Activation and Longevity Pathways:

Sirtuins, a family of proteins associated with longevity, emerge as active actors in the fasting-longevity association. Intermittent fasting stimulates the activation of sirtuins, putting in motion a cascade of events leading to increased cellular longevity. These proteins serve a critical role in the control of metabolic pathways, DNA repair, and stress responses, together supporting cellular resilience and possible lifespan. The complicated interaction between fasting and sirtuins demonstrates a dynamic link that goes beyond immediate health advantages, going into the realm of cellular longevity.

**8. Integration with Caloric Restriction Theories:**

Intermittent fasting's effects on lifespan mimic those reported in calorie restriction research. While not a rigorous calorie restriction, fasting causes a comparable hormetic stress response. This stress induces cellular changes that accord with the hypotheses arguing that lowering total calorie intake may lengthen longevity. The complicated dance between food scarcity, cellular resilience, and the possibility of greater longevity placed intermittent fasting in the lineage of treatments addressing the fundamental linkages between diet, metabolism, and lifespan extension.

In essence, this part unravels a tapestry of interrelated systems, crafting a story that frames intermittent fasting not just as a tool for immediate health advantages but also as a possible ally in the search for a longer, better life. From cellular rejuvenation and oxidative stress mitigation to inflammation management, repair process augmentation, and the activation of longevity pathways, intermittent fasting presents itself as a complete and sophisticated approach impacting the aging process.

# Chapter 4

# Tailoring Your Fasting Style: Crafting a Personalized Approach to Intermittent Fasting

Embarking on the path of intermittent fasting demands more than simply subscribing to a one-size-fits-all strategy. Chapter 4 dives into the art of customizing your fasting style, highlighting the necessity of building a tailored strategy that corresponds with individual tastes, objectives, and lifestyles. Let's uncover the deep aspects of this chapter, investigating each feature in depth.

## 1. Understanding the Diversity of Intermittent Fasting Patterns:

The journey into intermittent fasting exposes a spectrum of fasting patterns, each with its own distinct qualities and advantages. From the commonly used 16:8 strategy, combining a 16-hour fasting window and an 8-hour eating window, to more rigorous methods like One Meal A Day (OMAD,) where all daily calories are ingested during a single meal, the chapter gives a full overview. Readers get insights into the flexibility inherent in intermittent fasting, allowing them to adopt a fasting schedule that resonates with their daily routine and matches their health objectives.

## 2. Crafting Your Eating Window:

Crafting a tailored strategy includes a comprehensive study of the eating window. The chapter instructs readers on how to pick the length of their eating time depending on their lifestyle and preferences. Whether going for a condensed eating window, such as a four-hour period, or a more extensive interval, people find how to modify their eating windows to match their daily activities. This customization not only promotes adherence to intermittent fasting but also guarantees that the selected pattern effortlessly fits into their particular routine.

### 3. Personality Styles and Fasting Compatibility:

Recognizing the various characters of people, the chapter discusses how personality types play a key influence in fasting compatibility. Different people may find various fasting patterns more acceptable depending on their intrinsic preferences, habits, and psychological dispositions. By knowing their personality characteristics, readers may adjust their fasting method to accord harmoniously with their particular qualities. Whether someone is a diligent planner or a spontaneous adventurer, the chapter gives ideas on adopting a fasting schedule that matches unique personalities.

## 4. Thirty Days Fast Start: Personalized Guides for Different Personality Styles:

The chapter exposes a practical and individualized method with a thirty-day quick-start guide. Tailored to diverse personality kinds, these guidelines give step-by-step directions, ideas, and insights to help folks begin the intermittent fasting journey. For the analytical planner, the guide may stress comprehensive food preparation and scheduling, while for the spontaneous explorer, flexibility and adaptability take center stage. By delivering individualized instructions, the chapter guarantees that readers have a bespoke roadmap for their particular journey, creating a happy and empowered entry into intermittent fasting.

**5. Tweaking for Ease and Long-Term Sustainability:**

Recognizing that the intermittent fasting experience is dynamic and ever-evolving, the chapter finishes with advice on altering your fasting method for ease and long-term sustainability. Understanding that flexibility is important to prolonged success, readers learn how to make modifications based on growing tastes, lifestyle changes, and continual input from their bodies. This focus on adaptation guarantees that intermittent fasting becomes not simply a short experiment but a sustainable and vital element of one's lifestyle, promoting long-term health and well-being.

In essence, Chapter 4 provides a complete guide to navigating the diverse tapestry of intermittent fasting techniques. By encouraging individuals to embrace the diversity of patterns, tailor their approach to match personal preferences, and embark on a personalized fasting journey, this chapter ensures that intermittent fasting becomes a deeply personalized and empowering experience seamlessly integrated into the fabric of individual lifestyles and health goals.

# Understanding Different Intermittent Fasting Patterns: Navigating the Diverse Landscape

Intermittent fasting is a multifaceted area with a number of patterns, each bringing specific benefits. Delving further into various intermittent fasting strategies gives a full insight, enabling the selection of a strategy that harmonizes with individual lifestyles and health ambitions.

**1. The 16:8 Method:**

**Description:** This strategy entails fasting for 16 hours every day, followed by an 8-hour eating window.

**Benefits:** Beyond simplifying everyday meals, the 16:8 technique aids weight control by boosting fat usage during the fasting time. It increases insulin sensitivity and is vital for metabolic health.

## 2. One Meal A Day (OMAD):

**Description:** OMAD condenses daily calorie consumption into a single meal, often within a one-hour timeframe.

**Advantages:** OMAD simplifies meal planning, delivering possible advantages including greater fat reduction, better mental clarity, and metabolic efficiency.

**3. 5:2 Diet:**

**Description:** This strategy comprises regular eating for five days and reducing caloric intake to roughly 500-600 calories on two non-consecutive days.

**Benefits:** The 5:2 diet gives flexibility, supports weight reduction, and may enhance metabolic health via occasional calorie restriction.

**4. Eat-Stop-Eat:**

**Description:** Incorporating 24-hour fasting periods once or twice weekly, with no calorie intake during fasting.

**Benefits:** Eat-Stop-Eat improves fat reduction, increases cellular repair processes via autophagy, and may contribute to lifespan.

**5. Alternate-Day Fasting:**

**Description:** Alternating between normal eating days and fasting days with either nil or limited calorie intake.

**Benefits:** This strategy promotes weight reduction, improves heart health indicators, and may minimize the risk of chronic illnesses by offering regular intervals of metabolic rest.

## 6. Warrior Diet:

**Description:** Involves taking little portions of fresh fruits and vegetables throughout the day, followed by one huge meal at night.

**Benefits:** The Warrior Diet improves fat reduction, aligns with circadian cycles, and enhances mental clarity, giving a unique approach to intermittent fasting.

## 7. Extended Fasting (24-72 hours):

**Description:** Engaging in lengthier fasting durations, spanning from 24 to 72 hours, sometimes undertaken for deeper autophagy and metabolic advantages.

**Benefits:** Extended fasting promotes autophagy, encourages fat adaption, and may improve insulin sensitivity, delivering a more significant physiological effect.

## Choosing the Right Pattern for You

Understanding these patterns helps people to adjust their strategy depending on personal preferences, daily routines, and health objectives. Factors like as lifestyle, psychological temperament, and long-term sustainability play important roles in choosing the most effective intermittent fasting approach. Experimentation with varied patterns helps people examine how their bodies behave and select the technique that corresponds with their personal demands.

In summary, grasping the different topographies of intermittent fasting patterns helps as a compass for picking a method that not only accomplishes health objectives but also fits effortlessly into individual lives, creating sustained and successful intermittent fasting trips.

# Exploring Various Fasting Ratios: Navigating the Rich Tapestry of Intermittent Fasting Strategies.

Intermittent fasting, a comprehensive approach to dietary patterns, provides a range of fasting ratios, each having a distinct set of advantages. This explanation digs into the subtleties of common fasting ratios, including 16:8, OMAD, 5:2, and more, giving a complete guide to help you understand and pick an intermittent fasting approach that works smoothly with your health objectives and lifestyle.

**1. 16:8 Method:**

**Description:** This approach entails a daily fasting phase of 16 hours, followed by an 8-hour eating window.

**Benefits:** Beyond its simplicity, the 16:8 approach functions as an efficient strategy for weight control by improving fat use during fasting hours. It also boosts insulin sensitivity, a vital aspect of metabolic health, making it accessible for persons with diverse schedules.

## 2. One Meal A Day (OMAD):

**Description:** OMAD condenses daily calorie consumption into one meal, often taken within a one-hour timeframe.

**Benefits:** OMAD streamlines meal planning, perhaps supporting higher fat reduction, enhanced mental clarity, and efficient metabolic efficiency. The longer fasting phase increases metabolic flexibility and may boost cellular repair processes.

### 3. 5:2 Diet:

**Description:** Involves normal eating for five days and reducing caloric intake to roughly 500-600 calories on two non-consecutive days.

**Benefits:** The 5:2 diet provides flexibility, helping weight reduction via occasional calorie restriction. Additionally, it may contribute to enhanced metabolic health by giving intervals of nutritional rest and cellular repair.

**4. Eat-Stop-Eat:**

**Description:** Features 24-hour fasting sessions once or twice weekly, with no calorie intake during fasting.

**Benefits:** Eat-Stop-Eat increases fat reduction, initiates cellular repair processes via autophagy, and may help overall metabolic health. The cyclical nature of protracted fasting permits the body to reach a state of deeper regeneration.

**5. Alternate-Day Fasting:**

**Description:** Alternates between normal eating days and fasting days with either nil or reduced calorie intake.

**Benefits:** This strategy assists weight reduction, gives metabolic rest on fasting days, and may enhance cardiovascular health indicators. The alternating nature inhibits metabolic adaption, boosting the efficiency of intermittent fasting.

## 6. Warrior Diet:

**Description:** Involves taking little portions of fresh fruits and vegetables throughout the day and having one large meal at night.

**Benefits:** The Warrior Diet improves fat reduction, aligns with circadian cycles, and enhances mental clarity. The combination of brief periods of fasting with a midnight feast produces a balanced and sustainable approach to intermittent fasting.

**7. Extended Fasting (24-72 hours):**

**Description:** Engages in lengthier fasting periods, ranging from 24 to 72 hours, sometimes done for deeper autophagy and metabolic advantages.

**Benefits:** Extended fasting increases autophagy, promotes fat adaption, and may improve insulin sensitivity. This technique delivers a more significant physiological influence, fostering comprehensive well-being.

**Choosing Your Fasting Ratio:**

Understanding these fasting ratios helps people to make educated decisions based on personal preferences, schedules, and health goals. Lifestyle concerns, psychological temperament, and long-term sustainability play important roles in choosing the best-suited intermittent fasting ratio. Experimenting with varied ratios helps people study how their bodies behave and select the strategy that harmonizes with their specific demands.

In summary, investigating the complex tapestry of varied fasting ratios uncovers a broad variety of alternatives within intermittent fasting. This thorough knowledge offers people the choice to pick a method that not only accomplishes health objectives but also easily fits into various lives, creating sustained and successful intermittent fasting journeys.

# Unlocking the Benefits of Shorter Eating Windows and Embracing Variability in Fasting: A Comprehensive Exploration

Understanding the intricacies of intermittent fasting necessitates looking further into the benefits associated with shorter eating windows and the transforming influence of injecting variety into fasting habits. This investigation attempts to give a complete grasp of the research underpinning these techniques and their numerous benefits to overall health and well-being.

**1. Shorter Eating Windows (e.g., 16:8 Method):**

Enhanced Fat Consumption: Shorter meal windows, typified by the 16:8 approach, stimulate a metabolic shift towards effective fat consumption during the fasting phase. This metabolic flexibility allows the body to draw upon its fat stores for energy, contributing considerably to weight control.

better Insulin Sensitivity: Limiting the eating window leads to better insulin sensitivity, a cornerstone of metabolic health. Reduced insulin levels during fasting encourage improved blood sugar management, possibly decreasing the risk of insulin-related diseases such as type 2 diabetes.

## 2. Embracing Variability in Fasting:

**Preventing Metabolic Adaptation:** The incorporation of diversity into fasting patterns functions as a strategic approach to prevent the body from adjusting to a set regimen. By avoiding metabolic adaptation, intermittent fasting retains its effectiveness in sustained weight reduction and metabolic health.

**Disrupting Homeostasis:** The body instinctively seeks stability and balance (homeostasis). Variability undermines this balance, requiring the body to adjust to diverse fasting durations and techniques. This ongoing challenge is crucial to enhancing the advantages of intermittent fasting.

## 3. Optimizing Cellular Repair (Autophagy):

**Improved Autophagy:** Both shorter eating windows and diversity in fasting contribute synergistically to improved autophagy—a cellular repair mechanism necessary for maintaining optimum cellular health. Autophagy includes the elimination of damaged cellular components, possibly lowering the risk of numerous illnesses.

**Prolonged Fasting Periods for Deeper Autophagy:** While shorter windows activate autophagy, adding prolonged fasting periods sometimes, such as 24-72 hours, allows for more extensive cellular rejuvenation via deeper autophagy.

## 4. Managing Ghrelin and Leptin Hormones:

**Regulating Hunger Hormones:** Shorter eating windows and fasting variations play a significant role in the regulation of hunger hormones. Studies show that intermittent fasting may lead to lower levels of ghrelin (the hunger hormone) and higher levels of leptin (the satiety hormone), leading to greater appetite control.

**Balancing Appetite Signals:** The purposeful introduction of diversity prevents the body from settling into a certain pattern, helping to maintain a healthy balance of hunger and fullness signals.

## 5. Improved Mental Clarity and Focus:

Steady Energy Levels: Shorter eating windows and intermittent fasting variations help to stabilize energy levels by guaranteeing a steady source of energy from both food intake and stored fats.

**Cognitive Benefits:** Anecdotal data shows that some people feel increased mental clarity and attention during fasting times. This phenomenon be connected to the body's dependence on ketones for energy in a fasting condition.

**Incorporating Shorter Eating Windows and Fasting Variability:**

Understanding the depth of these advantages helps people to carefully integrate shorter eating periods and flexibility into their intermittent fasting regimens. Experimenting with varied fasting durations and approaches enables people to adjust their approach to suit certain tastes, daily routines, and particular health goals.

In summary, the substantial advantages of shorter eating windows and the inclusion of flexibility in fasting patterns offer a comprehensive and dynamic approach to intermittent fasting. This technique improves the physiological reactions to fasting, supporting not just efficient weight control but also complete benefits in general health and well-being.

# Navigating the Significance of Adapting Fasting Styles for Varied Lifestyles: A Comprehensive Exploration

In the multifaceted environment of intermittent fasting, the fundamental relevance of customizing fasting techniques to varied lifestyles becomes clear. This section tries to go further into the major reasons why changing fasting strategies based on individual lifestyles is vital for creating effective and durable intermittent fasting journeys.

**1. Synchronizing with Personal Schedules:**

**Professional Commitments:** Individuals with rigorous work schedules or irregular working hours benefit considerably from implementing fasting techniques that effortlessly coincide with their daily routines. This synchronization ensures that fasting times merge effectively with work responsibilities, decreasing disturbances and boosting adherence to the selected fasting technique.

**Strategic Integration:** Crafting fasting patterns that harmonize with professional responsibilities helps people manage their workdays without feeling confined by their fasting routine.

**2. Accommodating Family and Social Dynamics:**

**Family Meals:** The adaption of fasting practices to meet family meal times is crucial for establishing a feeling of oneness during eating windows. Flexible techniques, such as time-restricted eating, enable participants to have meals with family members without sacrificing their fasting objectives.

**Social Activities:** Adaptable fasting techniques enable people to manage social activities without feeling constrained. Choosing fasting patterns that include occasional flexibility promotes a healthy social life while sustaining the overall fasting regimen, and supporting long-term commitment.

## 3. Addressing Health and Fitness Goals:

**Exercise Regimens:** The adaptation of fasting regimens to complement certain exercise programs boosts individual performance and recuperation. Adapting fasting windows to correspond with exercise schedules ensures that the body obtains optimum nutrients during times of increased physical activity.

**Weight Management:** Adapting fasting strategies depending on weight management objectives provides for a tailored strategy. Some people may choose shorter eating windows for calorie management, while others may opt for longer fasting times to enhance fat burning, illustrating the adaptability of intermittent fasting in addressing varied health goals.

**4. Considering Psychological Disposition:**

**Stress Management:** Acknowledging the influence of fasting on stress levels is vital for sustaining a happy fasting experience. Adapting fasting patterns to fit individual stress tolerance assures that intermittent fasting adds to overall mental well-being.

**Cognitive Performance:** Tailoring fasting patterns depending on cognitive demands acknowledges the diverse influence on mental clarity. Individuals engaged in cognitively demanding work may select fasting patterns that boost attention and cognitive performance, displaying the flexibility of intermittent fasting to individual psychological demands.

## 5. Enhancing Long-Term Sustainability:

**Lifestyle Integration:** Adapting fasting approaches to easily fit with varied lives promotes the long-term sustainability of intermittent fasting practices. Choosing a method that compliments individual tastes, habits, and commitments enables a successful and persistent intermittent fasting experience.

**Avoiding Rigidity:** Recognizing the possible problems of rigidity in fasting approaches, an adaptive strategy helps people handle life's volatility while preserving the underlying principles of intermittent fasting. This flexibility helps to continue involvement and excellent health results.

## 6. Tailoring for Personal Preferences:

**Food Preferences:** The adaptation of fasting styles addresses individual food preferences, ensuring that eating windows fit desired meal choices.

to a genuinely 'Clean' fasting experience.

## 2. Scientific Rationale Behind a 'Clean' Fast:

**Insulin Reaction:** Delve further into the scientific foundation for a 'Clean' fast, stressing how even apparently benign tastes may provoke an insulin reaction. Reference studies display the physiological responses to sweetened liquids, emphasizing the important relevance of purity in enhancing the advantages of intermittent fasting.

**Optimizing Fasting Advantages:** Explore the subtle ways a 'Clean' fast boosts the advantages of intermittent fasting. From boosting autophagy to supporting metabolic flexibility, readers will comprehend how removing external stimuli during fasting times ideally prepares the body for greater health outcomes.

**3. Navigating Nourishing Eating Windows:**

**Balanced nutritional Intake:** Deepen the research of nutritious eating windows by highlighting the necessity of a balanced nutritional intake. Discuss the relevance of varied food categories in satisfying nutritional needs and maintaining general well-being under the limits of intermittent fasting.

**Mindful Eating:** Encourage readers to adopt mindful eating techniques during scheduled meal times. Provide practical strategies for creating a heightened awareness of hunger and satiety signals, establishing a pleasant and conscientious connection with food that transcends beyond fasting times.

## 4. Crafting Personalized Meal Plans:

**Tailoring to Dietary Choices:** Guide readers in developing individualized meal plans according to their specific dietary choices and limits. Showcase the versatility of intermittent fasting, enabling people to relish a range of tasty meals while sticking to their preferred fasting regimen.

**Exploring Meal scheduling:** Delve into the strategic element of meal scheduling within eating periods. Consider elements such as training routines and circadian cycles, delivering practical insights for maximizing food absorption and maintaining energy levels via intelligent meal planning.

## 5. Sustaining Long-Term Success:

**Building Sustainable Habits:** Highlight the shift from a controlled thirty-day rapid start to the formation of sustainable habits. Provide techniques for people to smoothly adapt intermittent fasting into their routines, stressing the lasting advantages of regularity.

**Tweaking for Comfort:** Address frequent issues people may have as they proceed in their fasting journey and give practical suggestions for fine-tuning routines to promote comfort and adherence. Equip readers with the skills required to continue their intermittent fasting success over the long run.

## Conclusion:

As readers end their transforming journey through "Fast, Feed, Reaffirm," the mastery of a 'Clean' fast and nutritious eating emerges as the cornerstone of prolonged intermittent fasting success. This chapter not only prepares people with the information to enhance fasting advantages but also allows them to build a balanced and nutritious attitude toward eating. In accepting the ideas presented in this book, people start on a journey towards long-term health and well-being, reinforcing the transformational potential of intermittent fasting in molding a better and more resilient lifestyle.

# Chapter 5

# Understanding the Concept of a 'Clean' Fast

In the changing environment of intermittent fasting, the notion of a 'Clean' fast emerges as a core principle, necessitating thorough attention to the items taken during fasting intervals. This section digs further into the subtleties of what characterizes a 'Clean' fast, allowing readers a complete knowledge of the concepts that characterize this purist fasting practice.

**Defining 'Clean' Fasting:**

At its foundation, a 'Clean' fast comprises a regulated limitation of consumption of certain substances during set fasting times. The focus lies on refraining from anything that might possibly impair the physiological processes linked with fasting. Accepted alternatives often include water, black coffee, plain tea, and sparkling water, but all other flavored or sweetened choices are purposely barred.

**Navigating Permissible Drinks:**

This part navigates readers through the subtleties of allowable beverages, offering clarification on what is allowed during a 'Clean' fast. Detailed analysis of coffee and tea covers typical issues, helping readers know the subtleties of ingredients and possible consequences of fasting advantages. The purpose is to equip people with the information required for a fasting experience untarnished by drugs that can impair its purity.

**Avoiding Pitfalls and Misconceptions:**

As readers begin on their fasting adventure, this section serves as a guide to stay clear of typical dangers and myths related to a 'Clean' fast. It addresses problems linked to apparently benign things that might accidentally undermine the desired fasting condition. By stressing the necessity of rigorous adherence to standards, it emphasizes the concept that any departure from 'Clean' fast principles may jeopardize the effectiveness of intermittent fasting. cc

## Scientific Basis of a 'Clean' Fast:

A deeper look into the scientific basis of a 'Clean' fast offers a degree of insight for readers. This includes an investigation of the idea of insulin response, clarifying how even non-caloric tastes may induce physiological responses that may alter the fasting state. Reference to relevant research underscores the crucial relevance of preserving purity in enhancing the metabolic and cellular advantages inherent in intermittent fasting.

## Optimizing Benefits Through Purity:

Readers acquire insights into how keeping a 'Clean' fast enhances the multiple advantages of intermittent fasting. From encouraging autophagy, the cellular recycling process that rids the body of damaged components, to increasing metabolic flexibility and effective fat utilization, the emphasis is on the holistic benefits received from removing external stimuli during fasting periods.

In conclusion, a solid knowledge of the idea of a 'Clean' fast is crucial for those navigating the complexity of intermittent fasting. This information helps readers to make educated decisions during fasting times, assuring strict adherence to the principles that constitute a 'Clean' fast and, in turn, supporting the realization of the greatest advantages of this revolutionary lifestyle practice.

# Factors to Avoid During Fasting for Optimal Results

In the quest for the best outcomes during fasting periods, it's necessary to negotiate some elements that have the potential to impair the integrity of the fasting state. This detailed book elucidates the important elements to avoid, arming readers with the information necessary for a successful and effective intermittent fasting experience.

## 1. Caloric Intake:

Maintaining a real fasting state needs a strong commitment to zero-calorie consumption during prescribed fasting times. Even minor calorie ingestion, whether in the form of snacks, drinks, or additives, might induce an insulin response, interrupting the metabolic processes needed for fasting. This section stresses the vital need to stick to a rigorous zero-calorie strategy for sustaining the fasting state and optimizing its advantages.

## 2. Sweetened or Flavored Substances:

The categorical avoidance of sweetened or flavored substances is crucial to a 'Clean' fast. Despite promises of being zero-calorie, these alternatives might provoke an insulin response, undermining the desirable physiological consequences of fasting. This includes avoiding clear flavored water, fruit-infused teas, and diet sodas. Readers receive a sophisticated grasp of how taste, independent of calorie content, regulates insulin levels and affects fasting results.

## 3. Gum and Mints:

Even apparently benign behaviors like chewing gum or ingesting mints may add tastes that undermine the purity of a 'Clean' fast. The act of chewing alone may increase digestive processes and promote insulin release. This section highlights the necessity of selecting alternatives such as plain water or herbal tea to retain the purity of the fasting experience.

## 4. Artificial Sweeteners:

The possible metabolic consequences of artificial sweeteners, widely used as sugar replacements, are discussed in this section. Despite being low in calories, these sweeteners may affect insulin levels, urging readers to pick alternatives aligned with the principles of a 'Clean' fast. Understanding the possible dangers linked with artificial sweeteners helps consumers to make educated decisions during fasting times.

**5. Processed Foods:**

During eating windows, the focus changes to avoiding highly processed and refined meals for maximum outcomes. Prioritizing entire, nutrient-dense meals ensures the body obtains critical nutrients without jeopardizing the advantages acquired while fasting. This section encourages readers to take a conscious and balanced approach to meal selections, strengthening the synergy between fasting and feeding.

**6. Excessive Caffeine Intake:**

While modest caffeine use is normally tolerated while fasting, excessive intake might have harmful consequences. This section includes suggestions on maintaining a balanced approach to coffee use, including problems such as higher cortisol levels and interrupted sleep patterns. Striking the correct mix enables people to exploit the advantages of coffee without defeating the aims of intermittent fasting.

**Conclusion:**

Armed with an awareness of these things to avoid while fasting, people may navigate their intermittent fasting journey with precision, maintaining the sacredness of the fasting state. This information helps readers to make educated decisions, improve their approach to fasting, and uncover the entire range of benefits associated with this transforming lifestyle practice.

# The Role of Varied Fasting Patterns for Long-Term Success

Achieving persistent success in intermittent fasting rests on a deliberate and dynamic strategy that goes beyond a static fasting practice. Delve further into the detailed analysis of why adopting diverse fasting patterns is vital for long-term success and the constant advancement of general well-being.

## 1. Overcoming Homeostasis: The Body's Adaptive Challenge:

Homeostasis, the body's intrinsic propensity to preserve equilibrium, may provide a tremendous hurdle to prolonged weight reduction. Despite the metabolic benefits of intermittent fasting, the body adjusts to a steady fasting pattern with time. Understanding this adaptation challenge highlights the necessity for flexibility in fasting patterns to minimize the plateau effect and support continued improvement.

## 2. Switching Approaches: Introducing Novel Stimuli:

Encouraging readers to swap fasting tactics frequently, this strategy delivers fresh stimulation to the body. For example, shifting from a 16:8 fasting routine to an up-and-down-day method upsets the body's usual rhythm. This purposeful diversity keeps the body sensitive, preventing it from falling into a predictable habit that may impair the efficiency of intermittent fasting.

**3. Varying Eating Windows: Enhancing Metabolic Flexibility:**

Exploring differences in eating windows during the day adds to greater metabolic flexibility. Alternating between patterns like 19:5 on certain days and One Meal A Day (OMAD) on others promotes intermittent challenges, improving fat-burning considerably after 18 to 24 hours of fasting. This detailed understanding underscores the advantages of shorter meal periods in preserving metabolic dynamism.

## 4. Hybrid Fasting Approach: Maximizing Adaptability:

The adoption of a hybrid fasting method, embracing multiple fasting techniques within one's regimen, enhances flexibility. This may incorporate conventional fasting days, non-restrictive eating days, and occasional exploitation of eating windows. This comprehensive technique prevents the body from getting unduly habituated to a particular fasting routine, supporting prolonged efficacy and minimizing the emergence of plateaus.

## 5. Caution with Extended Fasts: Balancing Intensity and Sustainability:

While variety is valued, care is needed when contemplating lengthy fasts. Prolonged periods without calorie intake might possibly lead to a slowing in metabolism, contradictory to the aims of intermittent fasting. Mr. This section gives subtle suggestions on integrating diversity without resorting to successive lengthy fasts, establishing a careful balance between intensity and sustainability.

## Conclusion: Navigating the Dynamics for Long-Term Success:

Concluding with a resounding focus on the relevance of various fasting patterns, this section highlights their crucial contribution to long-term success in intermittent fasting. By navigating diverse techniques and skillfully integrating diversity, humans may outwit the body's adaptive tendencies. This method not only promotes continuous efficacy but uncovers the persistent advantages of intermittent fasting on the route to enhanced health and overall well-being.

# Fostering Healthy Eating Habits Complementing Fasting Benefits.

In the complicated dance of intermittent fasting and nutrition, the intricacies of food choices play a key role in promoting overall well-being. This part uncovers the symbiotic link between fasting and good eating habits, giving readers extensive insights into building a diet that optimizes the advantages of intermittent fasting.

## 1. Moving Beyond Calorie Counting: A Paradigm Shift in Weight Management

Calorie counting has long been connected with weight control, but this part questions the accepted notion. It goes beyond the numerical focus, asking readers to evaluate the qualitative component of nutrition. Not all calories are created equal, and the emphasis moves towards nutrient-dense meals. By prioritizing the quality of calories above a simple amount, people may adopt a more holistic and sustainable approach to healthy eating that corresponds with the concepts of intermittent fasting.

## 2. Listening to Body Signals: Mindful Eating as a Guiding Principle

Mindful eating takes center stage as people are urged to reconnect with their body's signals of hunger and fulfillment. Drawing on a 2019 research exposing the effect of intermittent fasting on hunger hormones, ghrelin, and leptin, readers get a scientific grasp of how fasting might regulate appetite. This understanding helps people to read their body's messages, promoting a better connection with food that goes beyond the confines of discrete eating times.

**3. Addressing Nutrient Quality: The Role of Whole, Unprocessed Foods**

Nutrient quality emerges as a crucial component, arguing for a diet rich in whole, unprocessed foods. The debate expands beyond simply calorie limitations, underlining the need to fuel the body with critical vitamins, minerals, and antioxidants. Practical insights aid readers in adding a varied variety of nutrient-dense foods into their diet, harmonizing with the concepts of both intermittent fasting and general wellness.

**4. Shifting Food Preferences: Transformative Impact of Fasting**

Intermittent fasting is investigated not just as a weight reduction approach but as a catalyst for shifting dietary choices. The section dives into the ways fasting may modify people's desires, directing them away from harmful, processed options toward more wholesome ones. Understanding this transforming component of fasting helps readers adopt lasting dietary modifications for long-term health advantages beyond the immediate aims of weight control.

**5. Balancing Nutritional Intake: Mindful Choices During Eating Windows**

As people negotiate their eating windows, the attention extends to balancing nutritional intake. Mindful decisions during meals become crucial to guarantee a well-rounded distribution of macronutrients and micronutrients. This entails a careful approach to meal choices, maximizing the nutritional advantages received from both fasting times and eating windows. The section gives practical ideas for readers to manage their eating decisions carefully.

## Conclusion: The Harmonious Blend of Fasting and Nutrition

In conclusion, the section highlights the harmonious link between intermittent fasting and good eating habits. Moving beyond the limited lens of calorie monitoring, reconnecting with body signals, focusing on nutritional quality, and creating a change in dietary choices contribute to a holistic approach. This holistic integration not only boosts the advantages of intermittent fasting but puts people on a lasting and complete road toward overall well-being.

# Thirty Days Fast Start: A Comprehensive Guide to Intermittent Fasting

Embarking on a thirty-day fast-start journey is an intensive experience that integrates education, practical application, and progressive adaptation to intermittent fasting. This extensive handbook provides a comfortable transition into this revolutionary lifestyle, catering to diverse personality kinds and offering a holistic grasp of the process.

**Day 1-5: Introducing Intermittent Fasting Principles**

**Educational Foundation:**

Explore the underlying ideas of intermittent fasting.

Understand the notion of fasting windows and eating intervals.

Delve into the science underlying the metabolic alterations while fasting.

**Meal Timing Awareness:**

Begin recording your current eating routines.

Identify suitable fasting windows that coincide with your daily schedule.

**Clean Fast Initiation:**

Embrace a "clean fast" by ingesting just water, black coffee, or plain tea during fasting times.

Learn the significance of avoiding sweetened or flavored drinks.

**Day 6-10: Customizing Your Fasting Toolbox**

**Intermittent Fasting Patterns:**

Explore common fasting patterns such as 16:8, 18:6, or One Meal A Day (OMAD).

Understand the flexibility these patterns give for personalization.

**Tailoring to Your Lifestyle:**

Identify the fasting schedule that corresponds with your everyday activities and interests.

Experiment with various eating windows to determine what fits you best.

**Scientific Rationale:**

Gain insights into the scientific basis behind each fasting regimen.

Understand how these patterns impact metabolism and fat-burning.

**Day 11-15: Jumping Right In with a Structured Plan**

**Structured 30-Day Plan:**

Receive a thorough 30-day strategy geared to various personality traits.

Understand the trend from shorter to longer fasting periods.

**Meal Preparation Tips:**

Learn efficient meal preparation practices for maximum nutrition.

Explore dishes that correspond with your chosen fasting plan.

**Mindful Eating Practices:**

Integrate mindful eating techniques throughout non-fasting times.

Connect with the sensory experience of each meal.

**Day 16-20: Tweaking for Individual Comfort**

**Assessing Comfort Levels:**

Reflect on your experiences and comfort levels with intermittent fasting.

Identify any issues and any modifications required.

**Fine-Tuning Your Plan:**

Fine-tune your fasting regimen depending on your preferences.

Explore differences in eating windows for adaptation.

**Addressing Common Concerns:**

Receive tips on handling typical problems throughout the early phase.

Learn troubleshooting solutions for probable problems.

**Day 21-25: Reinforcing Healthy Habits**

**Tracking Progress:**

Establish a mechanism for monitoring your success over the 30-day trip.

Celebrate successes and milestones.

**Reinforcing Positive Changes:**

Reinforce favorable increases in energy levels, mental clarity, and general well-being.

Understand the holistic advantages beyond weight reduction.

**Connecting with Community:**

Engage with groups or support networks to exchange experiences.

Seek help and ideas from folks on similar paths.

**Day 26-30: Sustaining and Planning for the Future**

**Sustainability Strategies:**

Develop sustainability solutions for long-term intermittent fasting.

Incorporate intermittent fasting as a lifestyle rather than a temporary attempt.

**Future Adaptations:**

Plan for future modifications or alterations to your fasting schedule.

Explore continuous education and resources for continual development.

**Final Reflections:**

Reflect on the transforming journey over the previous 30 days.

Set intentions for keeping intermittent fasting as part of a healthy lifestyle.

This thirty-day fast start program offers a complete path for people to easily adopt intermittent fasting into their lives, supporting both short-term and long-term well-being.

# Final Summary

# "The Fast Feed and Repeat: Your Ultimate Guide to Delay and Avoid Denied Fasting Intermittently".

Embark on a transforming trip into the world of intermittent fasting with this book, precisely prepared to uncover the science, advantages, and practicality of this lifestyle. Divided into five chapters, each element unfolds to inspire readers in their search for comprehensive well-being.

## Chapter 1: Fasting Unveiled: The Power of Meal Timing

Delving deep into the science underlying intermittent fasting, this chapter elucidates the tremendous influence of meal timing on weight reduction and general health. It not only explains the nuances of insulin control and fat burning during fasting but also analyzes the body's varied reactions to diverse eating habits. By grasping the importance of time, readers get a foundation for the transforming journey ahead.

## Chapter 2: Fasting vs. Dieting: The Weight Loss Battle

In the conflict between fasting and standard diets, this chapter uncovers the unique processes that position fasting as a better technique for fat reduction. From suppressing hunger hormones to improving metabolism, it dissects the problems of traditional dieting and illustrates how fasting surpasses simply calorie constraints. Readers are taken through the nuances of the body's reaction, generating a better understanding of the usefulness of intermittent fasting.

**Chapter 3: The Expansive Benefits of Fasting**

Moving beyond the scale, this chapter explores the many health advantages embedded into the fabric of intermittent fasting. It becomes a voyage through the decrease of insulin levels, the prevention of Type 2 Diabetes, the struggle against chronic inflammation, and the discovery of the interesting relationship between fasting and lifespan. Here, fasting is depicted as a comprehensive technique, influencing not only weight but general well-being.

**Chapter 4: Tailoring Your Fasting Style**

Guiding readers through the wide terrain of intermittent fasting patterns, this chapter highlights the significance of tailoring fasting strategies to individual lifestyles. It argues for variety as a key to overcoming plateaus and sustaining long-term success. The chapter acts as a compass, helping readers to traverse the broad diversity of fasting alternatives and establish a sustainable rhythm that matches their specific requirements.

## Chapter 5: Mastering the 'Clean' Fast and Nourishing Eating

The last chapter crystallizes the trip by concentrating on mastering a 'clean' fast and developing good eating habits. It navigates through things to avoid when fasting, assuring the best outcomes. The relevance of different fasting patterns is highlighted for sustained success. This chapter provides a comprehensive guide, not just to intermittent fasting but to a lasting alteration of lifestyle and food choices.

**Thirty-Day Fast Start Program:**

Complementing the course is a painstakingly structured thirty-day rapid start program. From introduction to the basic concepts to customization, fine-tuning, and reinforcement of good changes, this program offers a path for people to smoothly adopt intermittent fasting into their lives. It goes beyond the physical elements, focusing on the psychological and emotional sides of the voyage. It's not a hard blueprint but a flexible guidance, respecting the uniqueness of each reader's road to integration.

**Conclusion:**

In essence, "Fast, Feed, and Repeat" is not only a guide; it's a full blueprint. It encourages people to embrace the advantages of intermittent fasting, not as a temporary remedy but as a sustainable lifestyle for greater well-being and longevity. Through education, practical insights, and a guided program, it acts as a lighthouse, directing readers towards a revolutionary and sustainable path of holistic health. The path toward holistic health is continuous, and this book serves as a timeless companion, ensuring your days are filled with sustenance, thoughtful decisions, and the affirmation of a healthy, vibrant self. May you step boldly into the future, empowered by the knowledge and practices learned on this transforming journey.